Acknowledgements

I'd like to thank my wonderful parents for their continued support in my adventures in life and helping guide me in the directions they have. Without their guidance I would never have been the person I am today. Their values and morals they've instilled in me to push myself to help as many people as possible in the best way that I can have been of great help in writing this book.

I'd also love to thank my wonderfully amazing wife for putting up with me through the duration of testing, implementing, and researching all of the topics that I've had to in order to bring this book to you. I'd also like to thank her for putting up with me during my periods of being grossly over-weight, under-motivated, and outrageously hyperactive and unable to focus at so many times. Her continued support through all the years has made this adventure possible, and here's to looking forward to all the rest we've got coming up.

And finally I'd like to thank you for taking the time to read this book – and congratulate you for taking control of your health – and your life. I hope you find it encouraging, informative, and motivating! You're absolutely capable of anything you put your mind to – and by taking the time to read this book you're on your way to learning how to use your Essential Oils in the best way possible to help you support your goals. No matter how far you've got to go, pretty much any obstacle you can name, I've been there too and understand how difficult it might be – but you can do it.

I'd absolutely love to hear your stories, struggles, goals, barriers you've broken through, anything you might like to share with me either on my Facebook page or website – I always enjoy hearing about it. I'm all for positive affirmations and would love to read/hear any that you are willing to share with me. Also, if you would be so inclined I'd love if you could post a short review anywhere you find the time to – and be sure to keep it honest. If you found this book helpful I'd love to hear and see it – and if you didn't I'd also like to know.

As the ancient Buddhist philosophy goes, "I can never be what I ought to be, until you are what you ought to be" – so here's hoping we can all reach our fullest potential in life, and help each other along the way.

Thanks again!

1

Important Notice

The information in this book is intended for educational purposes only. It is not provided in order to diagnose, prescribe, or treat any disease, illness, or injured conditions of the body. The author, publisher, and printer accept no responsibility for such use. Anyone suffering from any disease, illness, or injury should contact a physician or other appropriate licensed health care professional. The reader accepts full responsibility for the use of any and all essential oils.

Essentially

Fit

By Adam Ringham

TABLE OF CONTENTS

Introduction

This book will be a comprehensive guide on how to use Essential Oils in conjunction with your exercise program, as well as touch on many other subjects. There will not be time to go into all the different exercise programs and diet styles, as they are extremely numerous, and every person's body is different. There is no *one* way to exercise, but hopefully by the end of the book you will be informed enough to implement Essential Oils into whichever diet and exercise style fits your body, and your life.

As with all health related matters, please consult with your Doctor prior to embarking on this new health regimen. I am not a medical professional/consultant and cannot diagnose, treat or prescribe. If you have a health related condition, please consult your medical professional.

I will touch on more than just the use of Essential Oils in this book – but it is by no means a complete guide. -First thing that I like to recommend is that only high quality Essential Oils are to be used. For my personal use, I use Young Living brand of Essential Oils. Use of Essential oils that are from a trusted company is vital. Please make sure you have done your research to make sure the Essential Oils you use is of the utmost quality. There are many good companies out there, and there are a lot more that produce synthetic adulterated oils – these are NOT safe to ingest. Lab created does NOT equal natural – and even if it's labeled 100% pure, natural, and organic – these words really don't mean very much because you can lab create an essential oil and still call it "natural" – for the chemical formulas exist in nature – even though they are DRASTICALLY different. You can put gasoline into an essential oil and still call it "Organic" – as gasoline is technically and organic molecule. Also, many companies will use alcohol, other solvents, or "double distill" plant matter to obtain more oil out of a plant – and long story short, ruining your essential oil – and it is not safe to ingest. Hopefully you can see why I say make sure you can trust your company to get pure, unadulterated oils.

Treat Essential Oils with respect. A pure, Essential Oil is powerful both in good ways AND, if overused, in bad ways. Body damage can occur from a poor quality oil (as already mentioned) and/or from using too much. Start out slowly and listen to your body's response.

Throughout the rest of this book I will refer to "Essential Oils" instead of mentioning a company by name. I have had numerous personal transformations from the use of Essential Oils and want to share how they have help changed my life not only physically, but mentally and spiritually as well - this book will focus on the aspects dealing with physical transformations only. I have been in the most hopeless places, and have succumbed to the perils of "every day western society living". In college I was heavily involved in weight lifting and exercise, and like many people, got married, got busy, and got very, very unhealthy. I went from about 230 pounds at around 10% body fat, to finding myself weighing in at a whopping 305 pounds and losing nearly all of my strength. I did manage to lose about 50 pounds over the course of a year, but found the last 50 pounds nearly impossible to shed – until I found Essential Oils. So my entire weight loss was not due to Essential Oils – there are other factors that are extremely important such as diet, nutrition, and activity level. Each of these are JUST as important as Essential Oils – there is no such thing as a miracle cure or magic weight loss pill. You WILL most likely still need to do some form of exercise and/or dietary changes – but using Essential Oils can help make the task far easier. If that is what you are looking for – a magic weight loss pill - this book is not for you.

There ARE however, tools available that can GREATLY assist you in reaching your goals, be it losing a few extra pounds, being able to run a little further, a little faster, or adding extra muscle mass. To NOT incorporate Essential Oils into your life would to be greatly missing out. That is what this book will focus on, learning how to use the tools that are available to you to help you attain your goals. Take it upon yourself to learn not only how – but WHY Essential Oils are helping you. There are hundreds and thousands of products on the market, each claiming to be better than the rest. Each claiming it will give you an extra boost, each claiming to be "healthy". Well I've got news for you – most of them are none of the above. Most companies focus on fancy packaging, endorsing the popular athlete at the time, claiming to have the latest breakthrough, or just having a great marketing program. I've been there, I've done that, and I even used to work for a few of them. Don't fall for it. Take the time to research exactly WHAT is in them. You can learn anything you want to – if you just put your mind to it. Don't let anyone tell you differently, and don't rely on other people to tell you what to do. Not even me. There is no greater reward than taking your health and fitness into your own hands.

Chapter 1

Avoidance

"Health is not always about adding more – sometimes it's about taking things away"

It would not be fair for me to jump straight into the essential oils and their benefits, without informing you of many of the everyday things than can sabotage not only your health – but your gains (or losses – as in weight) and performance as well. There are so many everyday health hazards that it can be extremely overwhelming to start – so much to the point that it can stop you from even trying. I know – I've been there. It's A LOT of work having to pay attention not only to what you eat – but what you drink. My advice is just start somewhere. Nearly no one goes "balls to the walls" and does absolutely everything right away. It's a process, a journey, enjoy it. Your body will thank you. Not only will the process help you look better, but it will help you FEEL better as well. Your friends and family may end up calling you a crazy tree hugging hippie health nut – own it. Many will criticize you – while secretly wishing they had the strength to do the same. It's better to be hated for something you are, than loved for something you're not. People are going to judge you anyway, so it just as well be for things you are truly passionate about, things that matter to you – so let the haters hate and let the judgers judge. As a good friend of mine, Abby Huot says: "Don't drink the Hater-ade." Go on bettering yourself, not for someone else, but for you. Why would you want to get in shape, lose weight, or feel better, just for someone else? Do it for you!

I absolutely BEG you – look into all of the topics I will mention for yourself – and decide what's best for YOU. There is this magical auricle called "Google" that with a few keystrokes you will have all the information (and likely way more) that you could ever need. Don't just read one article on the following topics – read dozens – or more. That way you can make the decision that is right for you – not for somebody else – or because someone (like me) told you to. There is no greater mistake than to put the decisions regarding your health and happiness – into the hands of someone that bears none of the consequences.

If you've made it this far – then you can obviously read. If you can read, you can learn. Don't let anyone tell you that you can't. You can learn or do absolutely anything you put your mind to. You probably do it every day – be it looking up a tutorial, a how to, or a way to help yourself. You have not only the power, but the RIGHT to make decisions for yourself. It's your body, your mind, your life. Take charge of it. Take control! There's no harm in asking for help or opinions from other people, none at all, but ultimately the responsibility, the decision, and the consequences, are YOURS.

You are what you eat

I also encourage you to start paying attention to what you eat. While there is not room in this book to cover all of those topics – there are numerous books out there that touch on those topics. And if you need a little hint on which book to use, look for one that emphasizes healthy fats, green foods, and products that are Non-GMO and Organic. What we need to do is go back to eating actual food, instead of food like products. A great man Jack Lalanne once said, "If man made it, don't eat it. If it tastes good, spit it out". If you take a look at his numerous feats of strength, it will be very hard to argue with that statement. You've got one thing you take with you every day. ONE. It's your body. And it loves you. Love it back, take care of it - and learn how it works. All of these things cannot be done overnight, but one or two of them at a time CAN be done, and slowly over time you'll find that it just keeps getting easier and easier. If you start tackling one issue and making it a habit, pretty soon you'll find yourself not even thinking about it, because it's now part of your daily routine.

When you start paying attention to what you eat, you'll not only look better, but you'll FEEL better. And if your body has the nutrition it needs, Essential Oils will WORK better. All the oils in the world aren't going to be able to do much, unless your body has the tools it needs to operate correctly. Also, a person's body that is more acidic is going to need more oils to do the same job as someone who manages their body PH. And remember - change doesn't happen overnight. We didn't get into a position of being not as healthy as we want to be overnight, so it's not going to fix itself overnight. Just like you can't make a plant grow – all the yelling and screaming in the world, all the over watering, all the fertilizers, won't make a plant grow. The only thing you can do is give it the tools it needs to grow, and let it do it itself. Your body is much the same, you can't force it to do anything. You can only give it the tools it needs.

As we now continue into the part of the book you've been waiting for – how to use essential oils to assist with your exercise routine – remember that more isn't always going to be better. Yes they can certainly assist with weight loss, but don't take a half a bottle a day of grapefruit oil trying to boost your metabolism. All you're going to do is get a massive headache from detoxifying, along with possibly damaging your body as well. It's just like watering a plant too much, too much of something and you start causing damage instead of helping. There is no overnight weight loss solution, way to add extra muscle, or way to run faster. It all takes time, and your body can only go at a certain speed. Don't get frustrated, but rather – enjoy the journey. Learn how each oil makes you feel, how each food makes you feel. Really become curious about what you're doing, and how it's working. Remember that many times the few extra pounds you're carrying, is your body saving its life. When you eat lots of food laden with preservatives, pesticides, herbicides, and other things that really shouldn't be in your food, it can start to add up and become too much for the body to clear. Your body then has to quarantine these chemicals into areas of the body, and those areas are usually in the few excess pounds we carry around - places where they will do the least amount of damage. So many times, as we lose weight, we've also got to lose all the substances that we have built up over the years, and that cannot be done instantly. Give your body not only all of the tools it needs to recover, but also most importantly – the time.

Chapter 2:

Ningxia Red ™

Ningixa Red™ is by far my first supplement recommended for starting any exercise program. It approaches and helps with many of the roadblocks that those attempting to lose weight, gain muscle, or just improve overall health, with just one product. What is Ningxia Red™? Here's a peek:

Supporting Juice Blend

DESCRIPTION: Grape seed extract, Blueberry, Plum, Aronia, Cherry, and Pomegranate juices.

BENEFIT: Highlighting the supporting fruits found in NingXia Red is a patented grape seed extract that contain polyphenolic compounds that may help support a healthy cardiovascular system*. Additionally blueberry, plum, Aronia, cherry, and pomegranate juice contains naturally high levels of anthrocyanins and polyphenols, which block oxygen-based free radicals from damaging body tissues. Maintaining a diet rich in these powerful antioxidants is a recommended way to help prevent against a myriad of health risks and maintain healthy bodily functions*.

The new NingXia Red™, infused with the juices of these powerhouse fruits and pure, therapeutic-grade essential oils, has a Super Oxygen

Radical Absorption Capacity (S-ORAC) score that is 50 percent higher than the original formula, making it one of the most antioxidant-rich beverages available.

Wolfberry (Goji) Superfruit

DESCRIPTION: Wolfberry Puree (*Lycium barbarum*)

BENEFIT: The wolfberries sourced for NingXia Red hail from the Ningxia province in northern China. This superfruit has one of the highest percentages of fiber of any whole food and contains zeaxanthin—a carotenoid important to maintaining healthy vision. It also contains polysaccharides, amino acids, and symbiotic vitamin/mineral pairs that when present together promote optimum internal absorption. By using whole wolfberry puree—juice, peel, seeds, and fruit—Young Living is able to maintain more of the desired health-supporting benefits in every bottle of NingXia Red.

Pure, Therapeutic-Grade Essential Oils

DESCRIPTION: Orange, Yuzu, Tangerine, and Lemon Essential Oils

BENEFIT: The reformulated NingXia Red now includes seven times more essential oils! These carefully selected oils include orange and lemon, known for their ability to help maintain normal cellular regeneration*. They also contain high levels of the powerful antioxidant d-limonene, which is an important marker for bioactivity. Bioactives are natural compounds that work in harmony with your body to promote the healthy function of a wide variety of systems. NingXia Red also features tangerine essential oil, prized for its fresh flavor and its effect on maintaining cholesterol levels already in the normal range*. Exotic yuzu essential oil has been included for its uniquely delicious aroma, flavor, and high antioxidant content.

These pure and potent essential oils blend synergistically and deliciously with the other components of NingXia Red to support normal digestive health, healthy immune function, normal brain function, a healthy cardiovascular system, and much more*. No other nutrient-infused beverage can come close to the beneficial essential oil content of NingXia Red!

The Essential Oils in Ningxia Red also help increase your nutrient absorption. Just because you consume antioxidants and nutrients – doesn't mean that they #1:) Will be absorbed or #2:) Make their way into your cells where they can do their job. That's why Young Living has included numerous different Therapeutic Grade Essential Oils into this product.

Ningxia Red can also be used to help support body PH – which is extremely important. When your body becomes acidic, it has to work far harder to accomplish its bodily functions. Another lesser known fact, is that every single protein in the human body is negatively electrically charged – and that electrical charge has to come from somewhere. Body PH can simply be thought of as "how electric are you" – so when your body PH is within optimal range, your body has a much easier time assembling the key proteins needed to support muscle growth and normal body functions.

Numerous studies have also suggested that some of the ingredients in Ningxia Red can be used to support normal blood sugar levels – which is extremely important because Insulin is the most powerful hormone in the human body. Far above Testosterone, Estrogen, Progesterone, Pregnenelone, the whole works. So if your body has trouble using/making insulin – it's going to have trouble making the rest of your hormones as well. HGH (Human Growth Hormone) is also extremely dependent on blood sugar levels and sensitivity to insulin – but we'll save that for another chapter.

Also, the Wolfberries in Ningxia Red were found in studies to increase the time in which rats could exercise, decrease the effects of aging in mice, and suggest that it can be used to support eye health and immunity for astronauts during space mission. It also was shown to enhance reproductive ability in both mice and rats as well.

The final point I'd like to make, is that this proprietary blend also contains special forms of B-Vitamins that cannot be synthesized exactly in a lab, and B-Vitamins are what your body uses to make energy and get it out of the foods you eat. So if you're constantly tired, this is a great place to start instead of just drinking caffeine, because that is not approaching the problem, that is only covering it up.

It should be noted that when using ANY essential oil – the amount of water your drink is also of utmost importance. Many Essential oils help support an overall body detox, but those toxins don't magically disappear. They have to make their way out of the body somehow – and urination is one of the main ways your body accomplishes this. If you're not drinking enough water, your body has no way to eliminate these waste products, and you're going to have a harder cleaning yourself out. Long story short – drink an adequate amount of water.

Chapter 3: Pre-Lvl 1 Starter

Before we actually start getting further into the oils and using them with your exercise routine, I would like to suggest that your make it a point to learn every single thing that is humanly possible about each one of them. When you learn about each oil, you will learn how it can help you best. Each person's body type is different, and different things work better for some people than others. Try to keep a journal of which oils seems not only to work best for you, but how you used it, and when. This book will give you an overall guideline of where to start, but you will have to make adjustments to it as you go along, and find out which oils help YOU better.

Also one last thing before we get started, there will be different "levels" for implementing Essential Oils into your exercise routine – do NOT attempt to jump to whatever level you feel like right away. You absolutely must start at the first level unless you have been using them for a long period of time and understand them intricately. Rome was not built overnight, nor will your body be built into what you desire overnight either. It is highly recommended that you spend at least ONE MONTH at every "level" – if not longer. Do not feel discouraged if you stay at one level for a few months – there is nothing wrong with this. Attempting to jump ahead before your body is ready, will only slow your progress down. Eating "clean" and organic will GREATLY reduce the time that needs to be spent at each level. I suggest becoming "Powered by Green Smoothies" – but this book won't go into that very much, I'd just like you to be aware that the food you eat plays as much of a role in your goals (if not more) than using Essential Oils. Essential Oils are not quick fixes, or a "miracle-cure-all" – but they are powerful tools to be used that can help support you in reaching your goals. If you're looking for great recipes – there is a wonderful website called Food Matters TV - http://www.foodmatters.tv – you can go there and watch dozens upon dozens of excellent videos, get great recipes, and if you're looking for smoothies – just type in "Green Smoothies" in the search bar (or even just smoothies). Finally, I'd like to save everyone a little bit of money on something I spent quite a pretty penny on by doing it wrong over and over. Buy yourself a very nice blender. Don't skimp and get the Walmart special – or the latest super deal you saw on TV – get yourself the Waring MX 1200 XT 3.5 blender or a Vitamix (any of the models are fine) as well. My wife and I got a refurbished one directly from their website – 2 years later it's still grinding up nails (ok I don't really do that). Just don't do like I did at first and buy 10 cheaper blenders that burn out right away or don't blend very well – because you're less likely to eat your smoothies if your blender can't blend it up right and it's chunky, stringy, and you have to spend 30 minutes getting your smoothies to mix up correctly. Get something you can almost literally drop nails into and blend into powder (get a MAN'S blender VROOM VROOM!!!). I would also suggest that for the first while – skip getting a juicer. Not only do you have to go through a lot of vegetables and fruit to get the juice – you're leaving behind some of the most valuable parts of the plants when you do this. Get the fiber, grow a pair, and drink your smoothies! Now onto the Schedules!

Oils Introduced in this Chapter:

Ningxia Red™:

See Chapter 2

Lemon:

When we talk about lemon oil and exercising, we're using it to hopefully help raise your PH, increase metabolism, stimulate the lymph system, and stimulate the immune system. Citrus Essential Oils have also been shown to help raise Glutathione levels, the mother of all anti-oxidants. Also, lemon has been researched for its ability to help with the formation of red blood cells. This is important because red blood cells are used to carry oxygen throughout the body, and the more red blood cells you have, the better you can deliver oxygen throughout the body to muscle tissues.

Lemon is the first Essential Oil I will introduce can assist in maintaining body PH. PH stands for "Potential of Hydrogen" - and is basically a measure of how acidic or alkaline something is. Acids have a low PH – below the number 7, while alkaline is above the number 7. The scale goes all the way from 0 -14, with a 0 being extremely acidic (think of acids – hydrochloric acid, hydrosulphuric acid, hexofluorosilicic acid) and a 14 being very alkaline (think of AlkaLime (TM)). Your stomach uses an acid (hydrochloric) to digest its food, every time you find an acid it has a surplus of H+ ions (hydrogen), hence "Potential of Hydrogen".

Why this is so important, is because in order for your body to maintain a healthy environment it must be slightly alkaline – roughly 7.35. When our body drops below a healthy PH (or above even) things do not operate like they should. Your body will start to use blood sugar and creatine differently, it won't carry oxygen as well, and many other things as well. Another reason to pay attention to this – is because of Lactic Acid – a byproduct of exercising. It's the substance that contributes to making muscles sore. It's a naturally occurring product that your body makes 24 hours a day, but your body has natural mechanisms to clear it. Many oils and supplements can help assist with clearing and neutralizing it to help keep you from getting as sore so you can work harder, go longer, without the painful after effects being so bad. Also, when your body is acidic, your body has better things to do than build muscle or burn fat, so keeping yourself slightly alkaline is of utmost importance not just for exercising, but for overall health. It should be noted that the blood will almost always stay within a very narrow range of PH, roughly 7.35-7.5 – however, keeping it there if you're constantly eating foods or drinks that make your body more acidic – this taxes the rest of your body systems such as the lungs and especially the kidneys - not to mention it makes your body use extra vitamins and minerals as buffering compounds to neutralize that acid – energy that could be better spent in many other aspects of keeping your body healthy.

Lemon Essential Oil has a myriad of historical uses and is great for assisting with exercising. Not only can it help in keeping the body more alkaline, it's historical uses antioxidant, help with hangovers, relaxing, stress, unsightly veins, overeating, assisting with dissolving kidney stones, fever, supporting healthy blood pressure, dissolving cellulite, memory improvement, supporting optimal liver function, leukocyte formation, lymphatic system cleansing, red blood cell formation, energy, gallstones, and digestive problems. When we talk about lemon oil and exercising, we're using it to hopefully help raise your PH, increase

22

metabolism, stimulate the lymph system, and stimulate the immune system. Citrus Essential Oils have also been shown to help raise Glutathione levels, the mother of all anti-oxidants. Lemon has also been researched for its ability to help with the formation of red blood cells. This is important because red blood cells are used to carry oxygen throughout the body, and the more red blood cells you have, the better you can deliver oxygen throughout the body to muscle tissues. Also, Lemon Essential Oil helps the body better utilize ATP, more commonly known as Creatine. Finally, Lemon Oil can help assist your body with the buffering of Lactic Acid – the chemical in your body that is a natural by-product of exercising. It also is the chemical that makes your muscles sore, so the faster you can buffer it away, the less sore you are going to be the next day – and that's always a plus!

Valor (TM)

Valor (TM) is used to help support circulation and align electrical energies in the body – and there's no better place for that than the center of the body – the heart. All blood flows through here, and we can refer to the phrase "Heart Centered". Valor (TM) doesn't necessarily increase blood flow, but it does help blood cells flow past each other better. Think of Valor (TM) as coordinating traffic (red blood cells) better so the traffic flows smoother. As mentioned above with lemon – the more blood that is healthy that you can get to an area, the faster your healing can be.

Peppermint

Peppermint enhances blood flow by helping increase circulation through helping increase the size of the blood vessels and arteries. Think of it as adding more lanes on a road to help traffic through better – because if your blood vessels and arteries are constricted, blood cannot flow through as well.

Peppermint also helps increase the efficiency of other oils, and can help increase the efficiency of respiration, along with help increase intensity of nerve signals (strength). Remember, just because your muscle is there – doesn't mean that it will activate. You need your nerves to signal the muscle to activate, and the more powerful the nerve signal, the stronger a muscle contraction. Think of when you pick up a pencil, your arm doesn't fly to the ceiling and hurl the pencil upward, because you aren't activating your nerves as strongly than if you were lifting something heavy. When you're lifting something heavy or want a powerful contraction, Peppermint can help boost the nerve impulse (through the neurotransmitter known as Acetylcholine) so that your contractions can be more powerful.

Slique (TM) Essence

Slique (TM) Essence combines grapefruit, tangerine, lemon, spearmint, and ocotea with stevia extract in a unique blend that supports healthy weight management goals. The pleasant citrus combination of grapefruit, tangerine, and lemon essential oils adds a flavorful and uplifting element to any day, and can help with body PH management and the buffering of Lactic Acid (the by-product from exercising that makes you sore) along with the added support of spearmint that may help with digestion. Ocotea essential oil adds an irresistible, cinnamon-like aroma to help control hunger, while stevia adds an all-natural sweetener that provides a pleasant taste with no added calories.

Stress Away (TM)

Stress is a massive factor to consider when starting or enhancing a workout regiment. The stress hormone Cortisol is heavily involved in this chapter. Too much Cortisol is a very bad thing – and can come with numerous health complications. A little bit of stress is not a bad thing, but too much certainly is.

24

In today's modern world, we have no shortage of stress, and normally no shortage of Cortisol. While many hormones are dependent upon Cortisol to be made, too much of it can result in adrenal fatigue. If your body is too stressed out or Cortisol levels are too high, your body is not going to be worried about increasing its metabolism or adding muscle mass or gains in the weight room. Every time you work out, the stress hormone Cortisol is released. Every time your adrenaline gets pumping, you can be sure Cortisol is sure to be there too because adrenaline breaks down into cortisol. All of this ends up adding up on the body and taxing it heavily, so the more we can effectively deal with stress the better. This not only includes physically, but mentally as well. Outside of using Essential Oils to deal with stress physically, they can be useful mentally as well. When you are mentally taxed, your Cortisol levels will go up well, lowering your immune function, energy levels, and raising inflammation. I would highly suggest starting a meditation regiment, or other ways to mentally deal with stress, outside of just using Essential Oils (although they can be used to help mentally lower stress as well, and work amazing in combination with each other. Remember to make time for "you").

Contrary to popular belief, your body does not grow/heal in the gym, this happens when you are sleeping. If you aren't sleeping well, you aren't healing well, and your metabolism can suffer. Stress Away (TM) can help put you in a calm "Stress Free" mood so you can sleep through the night, and get the most out of your sleep. Your emotional state has a drastic impact on your physical well-being. Think of when you are stressed out at work, at home, with kids, family, and well when you exercise that is stress on your body too. A little stress is a good thing – but too much leads to adrenal fatigue and the feeling of being run down. Considering our modern day life style – a little stress relief probably wouldn't hurt anybody. I'd also like to quickly mention – and you should research this on your own as well – that doing excessive amounts of long cardio session is quite possibly the WORST way to lose weight – hence the cover of the book. The body will always respond with trying to become as efficient as possible, and if you're doing long bouts of cardio every single day – your body will do everything it can to make itself more efficient – which basically means it will slow as many of your body functions/systems as possible (metabolism especially!) to conserve enough energy to be able to do yet another long cardio session. It will do this at the expense of muscle mass, metabolism, digestion, healing, immune system function, brain function, you name it. I lost over 100 pounds not doing one single bit of intense cardo – so unless I'm just a freak of nature, you should probably do some research into that topic more. Also, if your trainer (if you have one) is insisting on you doing 45+ minutes of cardio a day 3 or more times a week – it's time to find a new trainer who has any idea what they're talking about. The other thing doing that much cardio is going to do – is raise your stress levels through the roof. So do yourself a favor – and skip the long intense cardio session. I'm not saying doing cardio is ALWAYS bad – I'm just saying it's an absolutely awful way to do anything but train yourself to do cardio (and not lose weight). There are people out there are training to do cardio, run marathons, triathalons, and that is perfectly fine! However if you're looking to trim up – large amounts of cardio are not going to be for you. A great replacement would be H.I.T. (High Intensity Training) and you should be able to find all the information on it online that you could ever need. Or even just start walking, just do SOMETHING – and you're on your way.

No matter what exercise or non-exercise program you're on, getting enough RESTFUL sleep is absolutely imperative. Have you ever slept for a long time, and found you were still extremely tired? If you keep waking up in the night, tossing and turning, this isn't good news. We all must get not only an adequate amount, but an adequate amount of QUALITY sleep. Sleeping for 12 hours will do you no good if it's not actual, restful sleep. The time your body does it's repairing of its self is when you are sleeping! Not when you're awake, that's usually when the damage is being done. The body needs time to repair itself, and if not given the chance you'll almost certainly doom it to bring in injury or illness.

Your body has its own internal and natural clock, that deals with awake/sleep cycles, and it's called the "Circadian Rhythm". It basically is regulated by the light and dark periods in the day (well along with many, many other things), and I mention this because of modern technology. I love the stuff unfortunately, and here's where they can affect the amount of sleep you're getting. When we stay up in bed, it's supposed to be darker to support your body knowing it's time to go sleep soon. The problem is, most of us are sitting and staring at this bright, white, stimulating light until we decide to call it a day. When doing this we can throw off our body's natural rhythm, so if we can try to avoid or limit the use of cell phones, TV's, laptops iPads, you name it, before bed – we can hopefully for FREE help you sleep a little bit better. It may also be helpful to have your phone charging across the room instead of next to your head – hey it's free why not try it, it can't hurt anything.

Personally when I am applying oils to help me sleep better, I like to apply them to my feet. I find that when I apply them there, the effects seem to come on slowly, are not as intense, and last longer – than if I apply them to my head or take them internally. If I really want to boost an oils effect before bedtime, I will put a little on my wrists and slowly inhale through my nose for a few minutes. And guys – there's nothing "manly" about not sleeping well. Even if you do smell like flowers, find something that helps you sleep at night. Unless, the manly man can't take it.

Cortistop TM (WOMEN ONLY) –

This is introduced in this chapter as an optional – but highly important topic. I'd mentioned above with "Stress Away (TM)" how excess Cortisol (from stress) really isn't a good thing. At all. High levels of Cortisol can shift the immune system away from metabolism regulation toward fighting inflammation that may not be there – but the "switch is stuck on" in your body due to high levels of Cortisol. Think of it this way – when you go exercise, your body focuses more on dealing with the stress on the joints and muscles in the body, due to either high impact or weight resistance – and focuses less on fighting off infections and recovery. If the chemical Cortisol is always being released due to either mental or physical stress, that's where the body can get "stuck". No matter if you're a guy or girl, please take the time to look into the effects of cortisol yourself. Ask your doctor to really explain it to you the next time you're in – or if you're comfortable look it up yourself. There are gazzilions of great resources from doctors on YouTube even about them. It's always best to ask your doctor – but it doesn't hurt to have specific questions to bring in to ask them about. It is not included in the workout schedules below because it is just for women – and you need to decide for yourself if you're stressed out or not.

Cortistop TM is a blend of Pregnenelone, DHEA, phosphatydlcholine (Forbes published a wonderful article on this ingredient I'm sure you can find if you look), along with therapeutic grade Essential oils such as Fleabane, Clary Sage, Fennel, Frankincense, and Peppermint to help increase effectiveness. Because of the possible hormone like activity of some of the ingredients – definitely bring your questions into your doctor on if this is right product is right for you. Who know? They may end up getting very curious about it you can figure out why that might be a good thing. Cortistop TM can be taken to help lower temporary stress once a day when you're going to bed (or an extra one right away in the morning for extra benefits) for 8 weeks, and then definitely discontinue use for about 2-4 weeks. Remember – you're not fixing the stress, you're just helping provide a little temporary relief from it. You still need to address the stress in your life other ways (*cough* meditation *cough*).

A note on Pre-Workout Supplements

The topic of pre-workout is one of my favorites to delve into, because I have personally have done it COMPLETELY wrong for a long portion of my life. If you are doing like I did, you will find yourself completely addicted to caffeine, stimulants, 5 hour energy drinks, red bulls, a massive myriad of poisonous cocktails to keep myself at a high enough energy level to go hit the gym. Then I'd take each and every supplement I found at the local workout supplement store in order to be able to push myself a little harder and a little longer. Here's the problem: I never approached why I had low energy (cough – NINGXIA RED – cough). The human body is much like a plant, under no circumstance can you MAKE a plant grow. The only thing you can do is give it the tools it needs to grow and thrive, it does the rest. The human body is no different. Forcing your body into having more energy does not work long term. Sure it might work for a little while, but pretty soon I found myself drinking 2 pots of coffee a day for years, then wondered why I'd get lethargic later in the day. Yeah, it's called caffeine addiction. And I'll tell you what – it was very unpleasant quitting. I personally have a hard time with this thing called "moderation", so I quit caffeine cold turkey – and holy cow did it suck. For at least the next 30 days I found myself sleeping for 10 hours a night, waking up exhausted, and then still needed 1-2 naps throughout the day. Don't be like me. If you need extreme levels of heavy metal music and every pre-workout drink or powder you can find, you're probably doing it wrong. I'm not saying a little bit of caffeine is bad by any means, but like I said I am just not good with this thing called moderation. Here's the good news, due to my mistakes – you now can learn from me and not make the same ones hopefully. And in the process, I found many other fantastic ways to make sure I had the energy to have an amazing workout, stay awake through the day, and not turn my body into a giant stimulant addicted poison filter. My pain – your gain. Oddly enough, I now even listen to classical music while lifting sometimes, because I no longer need that high intensity music to get a high intensity workout.

Schedules:

Pre-Level 1 AM:

1 Oz Ningxia Red right away when you wake up – and try to drink at least 8 Oz of water with it as well.

1 Drop Lemon - in 16 Oz of water – try to drink in the first few hours of your day. Lemon Oil assists in liver detox and body PH management, helps to clear toxins, and provides antioxidant support

Pre-Level 1 Pre Workout:

1 Swipe/Drop of Valor (TM) – 5 minutes before lift - rub in a clockwise circular motion in center of chest to drive the oil in.

1 Drop Peppermint Oil – in 1 Oz of water – consume immediately before your lift.

Pre-Level 1 During Workout:

1 Drop Slique (TM) Essence – In 16 ounces of water – consume during workout.

Pre-Level 1 Post Workout

1 Drop/Swipe Stress Away (TM) – Applied to wrists and inhaled for 30 seconds before bed.

Chapter 4: Level 1

Oils introduced in this chapter:

Lime

Lime Essential oil is much like Lemon Essential Oil, except it works in different body systems in slightly different ways than Lemon Essential oil does. They are very closely related, but if you smell them you can tell that they have drastically different smells, as well as interactions in the body. Although the uses are similar, Lime Essential Oil works on different mechanisms in the human body. Its historical uses include anxiety, support healthy blood pressure management, soothing broken capillaries, dissolving cellulite, lymphatic system cleansing, memory improvement, skin, tightening connective tissue, nervous conditions, and has also been studied for its effects on helping with the formation of red blood cells. As mentioned above, more red blood cells are very helpful for delivering oxygen throughout the body.

Grapefruit

Grapefruit is much like the other citrus oils, except it works in different body systems in slightly different ways than Lemon Essential oil does. They are very closely related, but if you smell them you can tell that they have drastically different smells, as well as interactions in the body. Although the uses are similar, Lime Essential Oil works on different mechanisms in the human body. Grapefruit has been heavily studied for its effects on appetite, metabolism, and its ability to help dissolve cellulite. One study found that participants that merely smelled grapefruit oil all lost weight and had their metabolism increased. They also found that it had an effect on appetite. Like Lemon and Lime oil, Grapefruit Essential Oil can be used to help balance PH. Historically its uses include appetite suppressant, cellulite dissolving, hangover, indigestion, normal weight maintenance, overeating, weight loss, lymphatic decongestant, headaches, water retention, jet lag, and cleansing the vascular system. Also Grapefruit aids in detoxification, especially in problematic cellulite areas, and can help assist in the buffering and recycling of Lactic Acid (the byproduct that makes you sore) – and adds additional antioxidant support to the body, and providing immune support.

Ocotea

Ocotea is extracted from an Ecuadorian tree, ocotea has the highest level of alpha humulene of any Young Living essential oil, which is a compound that helps aid the body's natural response to irritation and injury.* Ocotea also has natural cleansing and purifying properties. Ocotea also provides excellent support to the pancreas, and helps maintain normal blood sugar levels. Pounding large levels of carbs to spike your insulin to "drive nutrients in" – as you see many body builders doing - is not necessarily the best answer – try supporting your body's ability to make and use insulin instead.

Idaho Blue Spruce

Idaho blue spruce is an exclusive oil that is distilled directly from Young Living's St. Maries farm in Idaho. This incredible oil contains high percentages of alpha-pinene and limonene, with a pleasing evergreen aroma that relaxes both mind and body. The old legend also goes that animals in the wild would lie down under the tree for protection, recharging, and the rejuvenating effect it would bring them. The spruce tree was also used by the Lakota Indians to enhance their communication with the Great Spirit, and may help "open" the pineal gland. One of the most important things Idaho Blue Spruce can help with – is maintaining healthy hormone levels. Don't be surprised if after using it for a little while – you have a bit more of an urge to have more of that "special time" with your significant other. I'll let you figure out what I mean by that.

Life 5 (TM) (or other high quality probiotic) Probiotic

A high-potency probiotic, Life 5 (TM) (or other high quality probiotic)™ represents the culmination of years of extensive research. Life 5 (TM) (or other high quality probiotic) builds and restores core intestinal health by providing five clinically proven probiotic strains including two advanced super strains to enhance intestinal health, sustain energy and improve immunity. Life 5 (TM) (or other high quality probiotic) contains 8 billion active cultures and improves colonization up to 10 times. Nutrients are absorbed almost entirely in the intestines, and require a healthy intestinal flora (beneficial bacteria and fungus actually do most of this for you – and without them you cannot make B-Vitamins and many neurotransmitters – up to 90% of your immune system and neurotransmitters are made in the gut). So even if you're eating well – that doesn't mean you're absorbing everything – use Life 5 (TM) (or other high quality probiotic) to help enhance your gut health.

"Hey Girl – I hear you have a healthy intestinal flora" (insert picture of Ryan Gosling here). Guys, be sure to use that pick up line next time and see the reaction you get – it just might work, be sure to say out loud "insert picture of Ryan Gosling here" to increase effectiveness. Then strike up a healthy conversation on how up to 70% or more of your neuro-transmitters are made in the intestines (it's often called "Your Second Brian"), and up to 70% or more of your immune system is modulated by your gut as well. And if you really get brave, you can let your soon to be significant other know that the number of cells of bacteria outnumber your human cells by almost 10 to 1 (as in for every one of your cells, there's 10 bacteria cells (because they are much smaller!)). Then be sure to break out into singing Journey karaoke style or whatever else it is that you do so well. I mean, if the other person has put up with you this far, you can probably get away with doing nearly anything.

Terrible pick up line advice aside, the rest of the information is vital to your health - and well-being as well. We've covered a lot of topics so far, and just always remember, you can't JUST over-do one area and ignore the rest, it is far less effective than helping every body system. So as you go through the book, don't just do every oil listed in one section and none of the others – it will be a waste of your money. The goal is to make as little as possible go as far as possible. So instead of just taking all the stimulating pre-workout choices I'll be listing in one of the next chapter, choose one from each category (or a few at most to start with). That way you're supporting your entire body, not just "replacing a windshield and putting a spoiler on a smashed car".

Your digestive tract is where your body actually absorbs the food you eat. Absorption is key!!! If you're trying to get or stay healthy, getting the most out of your food is extremely beneficial. Along with modulating parts of your immune system, the digestive tract also makes many of the chemicals your brain needs to work. So if you're sabotaging your digestive tract with a persistent yeast overgrowth, sugary easily fermented foods, or ones high in pesticides/herbicides you're stressing your gut out. When the gut isn't in top condition, neither is your mind, or the rest of your body. Don't believe me?

Try getting even the simplest of task done when you're extremely hungry. Doesn't go so well does it? Take care of your gut, and it will take care of you!

Level 1 AM:

1 Oz Ningxia Red – with 8 Oz of water (either drink it straight or add to water, but be sure to have water with it to increase its benefits).

1 Drop Lemon Oil – Add to 16 Oz of water and drink in the first few hours of your day.

Level 1 Pre Workout:

1 Drop/Swipe Valor (TM) – 5 minutes before lift - applied to chest in clockwise circular motion to drive in.

1 Oz Ningxia Red – 5 minutes before lift either straight or in 8 Oz of water to help energize the body and sustain exercise longer.

1 Drop Peppermint – In 1 Oz of water and drink immediately before lift to get yourself fired up and energized further.

Level 1 During Workout:

Mix all 3 in 32 Oz of water and consume during workout:

1 Drop Slique (TM) Essence – Helps support metabolism and hunger levels, as well as tastes and smells good.

1 Drop Grapefruit Oil – Helps support metabolism, and the smell alone can increase metabolism and help decrease hunger.

1 Drop Lime – Also supports digestion and circulatory system, overall body detoxification, and can help support the metabolism, while adding additional antioxidant support to the body and helping boost the immune system.

Level 1 Post Workout:

1 Drop Ocotea – Hold under tongue for 30 seconds then swallow, and enjoy your favorite post-workout shake/meal (Green Smoothie!).

1 Drop Idaho Blue Spruce – Apply to insides of ankles at night (One Drop Total) to help support normal hormone maintenance in both men and women.

1 Drop Stress Away (TM) - Apply to wrists at night at bed time to help encourage more restful sleep

1 Life 5 (TM) (or other high quality probiotic) Probiotic – 1 Life 5 (TM) (or other high quality probiotic) Probiotic at night before bed

Chapter 5: Level 2

Oils introduced in this chapter:

Lemongrass

Lemongrass Essential Oil has historical uses support normal inflammatory response, revitalizer, tonic, vasodilator (for helping get blood moving more), healthy cholesterol levels, unsightly veins, tissue repair, connective tissue maintenance, fluid retention, lymphatic drainage, support respiratory function, and water retention. Lemongrass will primarily be used in assisting with exercising by helping to get the lymph system flowing/moving as much as possible. Blood carries nutrients to the tissue, while the lymph system is primarily for moving waste away from tissues, so the more we can get the lymph system moving to clear our waste and by products, the better your body is going to operate. Also – connective tissue is part of the lymph system, so stimulating the lymph system can help stimulate your connective tissue. Also did you know, the body contains nearly 3 times as much lymph fluid as it does blood!

Fennel

Fennel has long been historically used as an anti-spasmodic, anti-toxic, and expectorant. Fennel may also be used to help with normal formation of blood clots, bruises, colic, gas/flatulence, obesity, parasites, vomiting, intestinal parasites, menopause problems, urinary stones, PMS support, balancing hormones, and constipation. Fennel was shown in a recent study to help signal the immune system to stop attacking the beta-cells in the pancreatic islets, a key area for insulin production. Using fennel may help your body produce the insulin needed to regulate many key body functions such as blood sugar use. Fennel has been used for thousands of years for snakebites, to stave off hunger pains, to tone the female reproductive systems, earaches, eye problems, kidney complaints, and to expel worms. Fennel was also shown in recent studies to help with colic infants. Also, Fennel has been approved by the FDA as a dietary supplement.

Level 2 AM:

1 Oz Ningxia Red – with 8 Oz of water (either drink it straight or add to water, but be sure to have water with it to increase its benefits).

1 Drop Lemon Oil – Add to 16 Oz of water and drink in the first few hours of your day.

1 Drop Fennel Oil – Apply over pancreas before 2 biggest meals throughout the day to help support normal insulin levels and function.

Level 2 Pre Workout:

1 Drop/Swipe Valor (TM) – 5 minutes before lift - applied to chest in clockwise circular motion to drive in.

1 Oz Ningxia Red – 5 minutes before lift either straight or in 8 Oz of water to help energize the body and sustain exercise longer.

1 Drop Peppermint – In 1 Oz of water and drink immediately before lift to get yourself fired up and energized further.

1 Drop Motivation TM (blend) – Apply one drop to wrists, rub for 10 seconds, and then inhale for 30 seconds immediately before workout, with intention of being motivated not just in the gym - but in your life as well. Motivation TM (blend) helps enable a person to surmount fear and procrastination while stimulating feelings of action and accomplishment. It enhances the ability to move forward in a positive direction.

Level 2 During Workout:

Mix all 4 in 32 Oz of water and consume during workout:

1 Drop Slique (TM) Essence – Helps support metabolism and hunger levels, as well as tastes and smells good.

1 Drop Grapefruit Oil – Helps support metabolism, and the smell alone can increase metabolism and help decrease hunger. Also aids in detoxification, especially in problematic cellulite areas, and can help assist in the buffering and recycling of Lactic Acid (the byproduct that makes you sore).

1 Drop Lime – Also supports digestion and circulatory system, overall body detoxification, and can help support the metabolism.

1 Drop Lemongrass – Helps detoxify and support the lymphatic system.

Level 2 Post Workout:

1 Drop Ocotea – Hold under tongue for 30 seconds then swallow, and enjoy your favorite post-workout shake/meal (Green Smoothie!).

1 Drop Idaho Blue Spruce – Apply to insides of ankles at night (One Drop Total) to help support hormone production in both men and women.

1 Drop Stress Away (TM) - Apply to wrists at night at bed time to help encourage more restful sleep

1 Life 5 (TM) (or other high quality probiotic) Probiotic – 1 Life 5 (TM) (or other high quality probiotic) Probiotic at night before bed

Chapter 6: Level 3

Oils introduced in this chapter:

Thyromin (TM) –

Thyromin (TM) is a supplement designed to help support healthy thyroid function, maintain normal metabolism levels, and combat fatigue. More and more people these days are suffering from thyroid deficiencies, and keeping your thyroid healthy is also imperative to keeping your adrenals healthy (cortisol!). Thyromin (TM) is a natural antioxidant that contains Iodine, Potassium, herbs, amino acids, and the essential oils Peppermint, Spearmint, Myrtle, and Myrrh to help further ensure that it helps your thyroid function as properly as possible. If you're not sure if your thyroid is low – symptoms may include low energy, high levels of cortisol, slow (or fast) metabolism, and a low basal cell temperature (a body temperature below 97.6 degrees). Many people that have been exposed to high levels of fluoride experience low thyroid function, and Thyromin (TM) may help support the thyroid in returning to normal levels. Be sure to consult your doctor for advice on testing your thyroid levels if you have any questions.

EndoFlex (TM):

EndoFlex (TM) is the companion product to Thyromin (TM), and may help provide a balancing effect and support the entire endocrine system, as well as the pineal, pituitary, parathyroid, thymus, and adrenal glands. EndoFlex (TM) may also help assist with Hot flashes, stimulate weight loss by helping improve metabolic function, and help balance your hormones as well. Refer to Thyromin (TM) above to learn more about the thyroid gland and its function. EndoFlex (TM) contains Spearmint, Sage, Geranium, Myrtle, Nutmeg, and

German Chamomile to provide a myriad of benefits to the body, and is combined with sesame seed oil as a carrier.

Super C (TM)

Vitamin C is the quite possibly THE most important nutrient in the human body, because without it – it can take only days for the effects to take their toll. A disease that has been nearly eliminated now – Scurvy – can set in after just a few days of not getting Vitamin C. Vitamin C is also one of the molecules responsible for recycling ADP back to ATP (creatine recycling – also called the Krebs cycle, or Citric Acid cycle). Muscles cells, like all cells, use ATP (creatine) as an energy source. The total quantity of ATP in the human body at any one time is about 0.1 Mole. The energy used by human cells requires the hydrolysis of 200 to 300 moles of ATP daily. This means that each ATP molecule is recycled 2000 to 3000 times during a SINGLE day. ATP cannot be stored, hence its consumption must closely follow its synthesis. On a per-hour basis during intense exercise, 1 KILOGRAM of ATP is created, processed and then recycled in the body. Looking at it another way, a single cell uses about 10 million ATP molecules per second to meet its metabolic needs, and recycles all of its ATP molecules about every 20-30 seconds. Now you see why Vitamin C is so important – that's a lot of creatine to recycle! There are a myriad of different creatine supplements on the market, most of which are pretty much useless because they do not get absorbed, or fall out quickly into an form that isn't useable by the body (even in a matter of hours). What I recommend instead, is allow your body to recycle the creatine it already has as effectively as possible – that's where Super C (TM) comes in. Also Vitamin C is a wonderful free radical scavenger, along with helping boost immune function - and that never

45

hurts. If you do any sort of a detox, this is very depleting to Vitamin C, as it is one of the main nutrients used to produce detoxifying enzymes in the body. If there is one nutrient or supplement you are going to take while exercising, definitely do not leave out Vitamin C. Young Living's Super C (TM) also contains Bioflavonoids and electrolytes to not only help the Vitamin C get absorbed, but then help actually get into the cell and stay there. Young Living's Super C (TM) also contains Orange, Tangerine, Grapefruit, Lemon, and Lemongrass Essential Oils to help boost the absorbability and effectiveness of Vitamin C even further! You may also choose to use the Super C (TM) Chewable from Young Living as well if you desire.

AlkaLime (TM)

AlkaLime (TM) is a balanced acid neutralizing mineral formation to help assist with digestion and also help neutralize the environment that yeasts/funguses use to thrive in. The more balanced your body PH is, the less that funguses and yeasts can grow. Also, since every protein in the body is negatively charged, the more you can balance your PH, the more you can give your body the environment helpful to not only building lean muscle, but also helping to increase metabolism. Remember, your body has better things to do than burn fat or build muscle when your tissues are acidic.

Idaho Balsam Fir

Idaho Balsam Fir is mentioned here because of its ability to possibly assist with maintaining proper Human Growth Hormone levels and lower the stress hormone Cortisol. It's very stimulating and supporting to the pituitary gland. Many people believe that HGH levels decline as life goes on, but usually the levels do not decline with age, the problem more-so is the liver's inability to convert it to IGF-1 (Insulin Like Growth Factor – 1), so taking an HGH

46

supplement is not the answer. IGF-1 is responsible for carrying out the actions of the chemical message sent by HGH. Without a properly functioning liver, IGF-1 conversion does not take place near as readily and HGH has a limited effect on the body. Also – since Essential Oils are topically absorbable, Idaho Balsam Fir can be applied directly to a sore muscle to assist with healing. HGH is also primarily released by the pituitary gland, so the inhalation of Idaho Balsam Fir can assist the pituitary in functioning normally. Idaho Balsam Fir also works well with lavender and frankincense to support the hormones in actually getting into the cell. Idaho Balsam Fir may also help tone down muscle fatigue, temporary respiratory complaints, burns, coughs, wounds, sooth urinary complaints, may help sooth tendons, ligaments, and joints - and may also assist with back pain. Personally, Idaho Balsam Firs is one of my favorites for many reasons, and I was fortunate enough to go to the Winter Harvest and Harvest the trees for myself and make the Essential Oil all the way from cutting the tree down, hauling it out of the woods with horses, to chipping it up, to hauling it to the distillery, loading the distillers, filtering, decanting, and finally bottling it, the whole process – start to finish (I also slept in the wood chips one night – highly recommended!).

Motivation TM (blend)

Motivation TM (blend) is a blend of Roman Chamomile, Spruce, Ylang Ylang, and Lavender specifically designed to help one overcome the fear of achieving their goals and dreams. We often forget that the achieving of our goals has every bit as much to do with our mind as it does our body. Many times, fear keeps us from moving forward with our goals, because we can be afraid of what it would be like if our life were to change. As dumb as that sounds, we often fantasize about the things we'd like to accomplish – but at the same time in doing so our subconscious can hold us back, because of how drastically different our lives could be. Our life, routine, habits, and comfort zone will all be challenged to be something different than what they are now – which can be one of the biggest barriers in moving forward in achieving our goals. This is where Motivation TM (blend) comes in to give us the courage to move forward and face these challenges head on, and not be afraid of the one thing most people fear most – change. Motivation TM (blend) works best when smelled with intention of being motivated not just in the gym - but in your life as well. Motivation TM (blend) helps enable a person to surmount fear and procrastination while stimulating feelings of action and accomplishment, and enhances the ability to move forward in a positive direction.

Level 3 AM:

2 Oz Ningxia Red – with 8 Oz of water (either drink it straight or add to water, but be sure to have water with it to increase its benefits).

1 Drop Lemon Oil – Add to 16 Oz of water and drink in the first few hours of your day.

1 Drop Fennel Oil – Apply over pancreas before 2 biggest meals throughout the day to help support

Normal pancreatic and insulin function.

1 Scoop Alka-Lime (TM) – To help manage body PH more efficiently and create a healing environment in the body. Can be mixed with Ningxia Red or drank separately with 8 Oz of water.

1 Drop EndoFlex (TM) – Apply one drop over thyroid, kidneys, pancreas, or under throat vitaflex point under big toe in the morning.

1 Drop Idaho Blue Spruce – Apply 1 drop total to insides of ankles in the AM to help support hormones.

1 Life 5 (TM) (or other high quality probiotic) Probiotic – Take one capsule in AM to help support a healthy intestinal flora and maximize

nutrient absorption.

Level 3 Pre Workout:

1 Drop/Swipe Valor (TM) – 5 minutes before lift - applied to chest in clockwise circular motion to drive in.

1 Oz Ningxia Red – 5 minutes before lift either straight or in 8 Oz of water to help energize the body and sustain exercise longer.

1 Drop Peppermint – In 1 Oz of water and drink immediately before lift to get yourself fired up and energized further.

1 Drop Motivation TM (blend) – Apply one drop to wrists, rub for 10 seconds, and then inhale for 30 seconds immediately before workout.

1 Drop Balsam Fir – Apply one drop to chest immediately before workout – and to sore muscles as desired throughout the day.

Level 3 During Workout:

Mix all 4 in 32 Oz of water and consume during workout:

1 Drop Slique (TM) Essence – Helps support metabolism and hunger levels, as well as tastes and smells good.

1 Drop Grapefruit Oil – Helps support metabolism, and the smell alone can increase metabolism and help decrease hunger. Also aids in detoxification, especially in problematic cellulite areas, and can help assist in the buffering and recycling of Lactic Acid (the byproduct that makes you sore).

1 Drop Lime – Also supports digestion and circulatory system, overall body detoxification, and can help support the metabolism.

1 Drop Lemongrass – Helps detoxify and support the lymphatic system.

Level 3 Post Workout:

1 Drop Ocotea – Hold under tongue for 30 seconds then swallow, and enjoy your favorite post-workout shake/meal (Slique (TM) Bar/Green Smoothie!).

1 Drop Idaho Blue Spruce – Apply to insides of ankles at night (One Drop Total) to help support hormone production in both men and women.

1 Drop Stress Away (TM) - Apply to wrists at night at bed time to help encourage more restful sleep.

1 Life 5 (TM) (or other high quality probiotic) Probiotic – 1 Life 5 (TM) (or other high quality probiotic) Probiotic at night before bed.

1 Pill Thyromin (TM) – Take before bed to help support thyroid function.

Chapter 7 – Optional

Progessence Plus (TM) (women)

Progessence Plus (TM) is a serum that contains natural, fully developed micronized progesterone derived from wild yam root, along with the essential oils Frankincense, Cedarwood, Copaiba, Peppermint, and more to enhance absorption into the deeper layers of the skin where it can be picked up by the blood vessels and delivered to the body. Progesterone I a beautiful hormone that when at optimal levels can help with weight loss, reduce the risk of stroke and heart attack, hair loss, normalize sleeping, energy levels, abnormal blood sugar levels, thyroid action, acne (and double especially around the chin area), improve bone density, libido, cell oxygenation, decrease symptoms of menopause, backaches, temporary depression, exhaustion, and more. I would HIGHLY suggest looking into the FAQ's and books Dr. Dan Purser has written, they are amazing. Also it is heavily worth noting, that when you start using Progessence Plus (TM), many times your symptoms (acne, hot flashes, etc.) will get worse before they get better. Xenoestrogens as your body rids it's self of them, have to go somewhere – and the detox symptoms can be a little obnoxious. Stick with it – you'll be glad you did. Also I must say that this is NOT an artificial hormone, I am against using artificial hormones COMPLETELY. They are poorly assimilated by the body, and force it into a state it would not normally be in. Also – do NOT take Progessence Plus (TM) if you are on birth control or other hormone medications – they do not go well together. Once the detox symptoms have been completed, you will definitely thank yourself, and your body will too. Keep in mind, it may take 6 months or more of use before your reach the place you want to be at. If the detox symptoms get too much, just use less, or skip a day here and there. Pay attention to everything I'd mentioned earlier in this chapter – the more of the things I'd mentioned you should avoid that you haven't in your life, usually the longer it will take for your hormone levels to normalize (especially if you've been on any form of birth control). Lastly, I'll repeat it: Get Dr. Dan Purser's books (many times they are free) on progesterone (Progessence Plus (TM)), or at the very least read what he has to say quickly – the more you know about the product, the better you can make it work.

Shutran (TM) (men mostly, women too):

Shutran (TM) is an empowering essential oil blend that is formulated specifically for men to boost feelings of masculinity, confidence, and attractiveness. It is best used as a cologne, and there is absolutely nothing artificial or synthetic in it. Although this is formulated specifically for men, women may also get benefit from it as well. Shutran (TM) can be used to help get you through that impossible workout, or to help in the pursuit of that special evening. Shutran (TM) contains Idaho Blue Spruce, Ocotea, Hinoki, Ylang Ylang, Coriander, Davana, Cedarwood, Lemon, and Lavender Essential Oils. Men or Women – this is an excellent blend for helping balance hormones, to help get "in the mood", or to give that workout very special type of boost (plus you're going to smell amazing). Works well as a cologne or perfume throughout the day.

Black Pepper:

Black pepper helps to block the stress hormone cortisol, and can help increase nutrient absorption as well. All the nutrients in the world won't do you much good, unless you can absorb them and get them into the cell. We're constantly under stress every day, all day, especially in this modern world. The more we can do to help ward off the damages of stress, the better our bodies can heal and recover. Black pepper also can increase lipid oxidation (fat burning) while inhibiting lipid peroxidation (essentially fat that breaks down wrong). Black pepper goes well topically over the adrenal glands (middle of the back on top of kidneys), and can also be used in a veggie capsule. Black pepper is one of my favorites for helping to increase stamina, and I feel is good for those looking for long intense workouts (running, marathons, triathlons, or just long intense workout sessions). Black pepper has historically been used to help with temporary inflammatory conditions, catarrhal, spasms, stimulating the nervous, circulatory, and digestive systems, fainting, increasing cellular oxygenation, increasing energy, chills, loss of appetite, colds, constipation, coughs, poor circulation, poor muscle tone, sprains, neuralgia, flue, vertigo and vomiting. Works best when applied over the adrenals (kidneys) at any point in the day.

Aroma Siez:

The oils in this blend work synergistically to help calm the aches, pains, and general soreness of temporary spastic muscles. With Basil, Marjoram, Lavender, Peppermint, and Cypress – this is a wonderful companion oil to have for anyone that has worked their muscles hard and gotten them sore. Works best when applied anytime throughout the day specifically to sore muscles.

Ultra Young (TM) + Spray

Ultra Young (TM) + Spray is NOT an HGH supplement, just like Idaho Balsam Fir. What it is however, is a unique product that helps allow your body to use the HGH you produce naturally more efficiently. It also is a delivery system that works to be absorbed through the Oral Mucosa (which can greatly enhance the amount of supplements delivered over a pill or capsule form) that then is protected from rapid first pass metabolism by the liver, helping to keep the ingredients more intact. It is also worth noting that HGH conversion works best when your blood sugars are low, so fasting is exceptionally beneficial, not only with the use of this supplement, but in general. It is best to avoid eating for around 2-4 hours around the time that you are going to use this supplement. Ultra Young (TM) Plus also contains Ningxia Wolfberries for their Insulin supporting action, DHEA (since the production of this usually declines after your 20s), and may other supportive vitamins and essential oils. Both Ultra Young (TM) Plus and Idaho Balsam Fir are included in the "insulin" section of the book because of HGH's relation to insulin (hence, Insulin Like Growth Factor – 1 conversion), and it's abilities to be enhanced by fasting and low blood sugars. Ultra Young (TM) + is best sprayed on the cheeks and roof of the mouth for enhanced absorption, and avoid spraying on the tongue to decrease saliva production. It is also worth noting that HGH works best when the liver, pancreas, and thyroid are all functioning normally, so it may be beneficial to use both Ultra Young (TM) + and Idaho Balsam Fir with oils and supplements that support these organs, such as Thyromin (TM) and JuvaTone. Remember that stimulating the pituitary alone is a very one sided approach – which is just another way of saying you're only setting yourself up for failure by trying to overcompensate in one area, and not looking at the body like an entire machine. But instead, supporting the entire system, instead of just "making the tires bigger". It is also worth noting that HGH drastically raises inflammatory cytokines, and using essential oils to help neutralize them can help greatly enhances your body's ability to grow, recover, and boost its metabolism.

Chapter 8 – Summing it up

Hopefully you're not too overwhelmed by all of the different options you have to use Essential Oils during the course of your workout – because there are a lot of them! And by no means is this a perfect fit for every single person – this is only a guide to get you started. Later on I'll have another book on how increase muscle mass and endurance, but unless you can get to at least level 2 in this book – there's no way that you can get started with the further levels without horrid detox symptoms (such as headache, excessive perspiration, or worse). Integrating Essential Oils into your lifestyle and workout regiment requires time and effort, it works best if you slowly replace the supplements that are chemically laden poison with those that are natural, and don't force the body – that instead give it the tools it needs to do its job. It's also worth noting – that even one night of drinking with your friends, one meal of eating out at a fast food restaurant, can set you back a week or more in your attempts to advance in the levels. Also be sure to LISTEN TO YOUR BODY. There is a such thing as too much of a good thing – and if you're feeling tired, sluggish, sick, run down, or just generally not well – back off on the oils. To get to level 3 you honestly should plan on it taking a year or more. Don't shoot the messenger, but due to our lifestyles that have become common place – it will take time to adjust and clean the body out. Just like bringing your car to a mechanic – he's going to need to order parts, take the broken ones off, and put the new ones on – your body is a far more complex machine with even more complicated interwoven systems that take time to heal and regenerate. Your body is the most luxury of all expensive sports cars that you can imagine, and is worth far more.

And the thing is – you don't just get to trade your body in for a new one – take the time to take care of the ONE thing that is not replaceable in your life – as much as you do the things that can be replaced. Because after all – the first wealth is health. How much time do you spend washing your car, cleaning your house, mowing your lawn, organizing the basement, picking out what clothes or cell phone to buy, figuring out what to post on Facebook, picking the perfect response text, planning a night with friends, watching TV, checking your email, cutting coupons, or finding the lowest gas prices? Do you think that you could maybe – just maybe – limit your sitting, eating, sleeping, and all those other things to just 23.5 hours a day? I bet you can.

The best suggestion I have in getting started – is just jump in. Start with the Pre-Level One schedule, and give it a little time. Also every time you use an Essential Oil – look up what is for and WHY you're using it every time you use it, because if you understand why you're using it – you can get more out of them – and be able to tell people about it easier from memory in case they ask. A super handy reference is "The Essential Oil Desk Reference" that can be purchased many places online – and take the time to review every oil or supplement you're going to use every time you use it. After a little while it'll become second nature, and you'll understand more of why you're using it.

It also wouldn't hurt to keep a journal. Be sure to put in what you took, what you lifted, and most importantly how you feel. Don't waste your time looking at the scale 10 times a day – I suggest throwing the thing away and just paying attention to how your clothes fit. Women – don't be scared of a little muscle mass. Lifting weights isn't going to make you a hulk, and every pound of muscle burns 10x more calories than a pound of fat, just sitting there. Also when you gain more muscle, you're adding protection to your body to bumps, bruises, slips, falls, and everyday life occurrences. Do your best to watch what you eat as well (I highly suggest doing a little Google research on "grains are not a health food") – because the less healthy you eat – the less effect Essential Oils will have. It's a partnership – Essential Oils are the right hand, and your food is the left hand – you can accomplish a lot more when you're using both hands (try to lift something with just one hand – you'll find it's a lot more difficult and your balance will be thrown off).

You also could look into hiring a personal trainer (one that doesn't have you doing hours of cardio all the time – because that won't do you any good) – because who knows? They might end up being an Essential Oil client of yours after a little while (trainers are always looking for ways to help their clients – perhaps they'd be interested in a copy of this book...).

Lastly and MOST importantly – have fun with it. Don't take exercising as a chore – instead start with positive affirmations that you are going to have fun today integrating Essential Oils into your workout. You don't have to start balls to the walls – just start somewhere. Maybe you've got a favorite TV show you watch – throw it on with your iPad or whatever you have and watch it while you walk or ride an exercise bike (I personally like the elliptical machines due to the low impact and whole body workout integration).

Don't waste time comparing yourself to other people – because they are not you. It would be like trying to compare apples and nails – under no circumstance do you fit in any of the same categories someone else does. Your body is different, your mind is different, and every single thing about you is completely different than the person next to you – why on earth would you try to compare yourself to them? That is the surest way to set yourself up for failure – comparing yourself to someone else.

Try writing on the mirror that you look at every day your goals, your dreams, your aspirations, and a reminder that you love yourself. Your body loves you, love it back. Another great step that I highly recommend to EVERYBODY – cancel your cable TV. Not only is it expensive, but all it is going to do is end up making you waste time if you keep it. Use the money that you would have spent on the cable bill, on yourself and your health instead. 50% of your favorite TV show is commercials telling you to buy this, have that, and compare yourself to someone that has been photoshopped into something they're not. Don't live a lie - live you, do you, be you. Do your best every day, and understand that you will not be perfect every day. Forgive yourself – as the famous Nikola Tesla once said "I've never failed, I've only found 900 ways that didn't work".

The only difference between a master and a beginner is that the master has "failed" more times than the beginner has even attempted (remember not failed – just found ways that didn't work). Try to look back a year, a month, or even a week – do you really remember the times something didn't work? Probably not – but can you remember the times you did succeed? Focus on those, take time to identify the times you did succeed and cherish them, celebrate them. Yell them at your husband or wife (or cat) "I SUCCEEDED!!!" and watch their reaction – it will probably be hilarious. A year from now you'll be glad you started today – start a new chapter in the story called "Your Life", write a new ending, do something you've never done, and change the way you look at today, every day, and most importantly yourself.

Because when you change the way you look at things – the things you look at change...

Get Oiled Up!

Schedules:

Pre-Level 1 AM:

1 Oz Ningxia Red right away when you wake up – and try to drink at least 8 Oz of water with it as well.

1 Drop Lemon - in 16 Oz of water – try to drink in the first few hours of your day. Lemon Oil assists in liver detox and body PH management, helps to clear toxins, and provides antioxidant support

Pre-Level 1 Pre Workout:

1 Swipe/Drop of Valor (TM) – 5 minutes before lift - rub in a clockwise circular motion in center of chest to drive the oil in.

1 Drop Peppermint Oil – in 1 Oz of water – consume immediately before your lift.

Pre-Level 1 During Workout:

1 Drop Slique (TM) Essence – In 16 ounces of water – consume during workout.

Pre-Level 1 Post Workout

1 Drop/Swipe Stress Away (TM) – Applied to wrists and inhaled for 30 seconds before bed.

Level 1 AM:

1 Oz Ningxia Red – with 8 Oz of water (either drink it straight or add to water, but be sure to have water with it to increase its benefits).

1 Drop Lemon Oil – Add to 16 Oz of water and drink in the first few hours of your day.

Level 1 Pre Workout:

1 Drop/Swipe Valor (TM) – 5 minutes before lift - applied to chest in clockwise circular motion to drive in.

1 Oz Ningxia Red – 5 minutes before lift either straight or in 8 Oz of water to help energize the body and sustain exercise longer.

1 Drop Peppermint – In 1 Oz of water and drink immediately before lift to get yourself fired up and energized further.

Level 1 During Workout:

Mix all 3 in 32 Oz of water and consume during workout:

1 Drop Slique (TM) Essence – Helps support metabolism and hunger levels, as well as tastes and smells good.

1 Drop Grapefruit Oil – Helps support metabolism, and the smell alone can increase metabolism and help decrease hunger.

1 Drop Lime – Also supports digestion and circulatory system, overall body detoxification, and can help support the metabolism, while adding additional antioxidant support to the body and helping boost the immune system.

Level 1 Post Workout:

1 Drop Ocotea – Hold under tongue for 30 seconds then swallow, and enjoy your favorite post-workout shake/meal (Green Smoothie!).

1 Drop Idaho Blue Spruce – Apply to insides of ankles at night (One Drop Total) to help support normal hormone maintenance in both men and women.

1 Drop Stress Away (TM) - Apply to wrists at night at bed time to help encourage more restful sleep

1 Life 5 (TM) (or other high quality probiotic) Probiotic – 1 Life 5 (TM) (or other high quality probiotic) Probiotic at night before bed

Level 2 AM:

1 Oz Ningxia Red – with 8 Oz of water (either drink it straight or add to water, but be sure to have water with it to increase its benefits).

1 Drop Lemon Oil – Add to 16 Oz of water and drink in the first few hours of your day.

1 Drop Fennel Oil – Apply over pancreas before 2 biggest meals throughout the day to help support

Normal insulin levels and function.

Level 2 Pre Workout:

1 Drop/Swipe Valor (TM) – 5 minutes before lift - applied to chest in clockwise circular motion to drive in.

1 Oz Ningxia Red – 5 minutes before lift either straight or in 8 Oz of water to help energize the body and sustain exercise longer.

1 Drop Peppermint – In 1 Oz of water and drink immediately before lift to get yourself fired up and energized further.

1 Drop Motivation TM (blend) – Apply one drop to wrists, rub for 10 seconds, and then inhale for 30 seconds immediately before workout, with intention of being motivated not just in the gym - but in your life as well. Motivation TM (blend) helps enable a person to surmount fear and procrastination while stimulating feelings of action and accomplishment. It enhances the ability to move forward in a positive direction.

Level 2 During Workout:

Mix all 4 in 32 Oz of water and consume during workout:

1 Drop Slique (TM) Essence – Helps support metabolism and hunger levels, as well as tastes and smells good.

1 Drop Grapefruit Oil – Helps support metabolism, and the smell alone can increase metabolism and help decrease hunger. Also aids in detoxification, especially in problematic cellulite areas, and can help assist in the buffering and recycling of Lactic Acid (the byproduct that makes you sore).

1 Drop Lime – Also supports digestion and circulatory system, overall body detoxification, and can help support the metabolism.

1 Drop Lemongrass – Helps detoxify and support the lymphatic system.

Level 2 Post Workout:

1 Drop Ocotea – Hold under tongue for 30 seconds then swallow, and enjoy your favorite post-workout shake/meal (Green Smoothie!).

1 Drop Idaho Blue Spruce – Apply to insides of ankles at night (One Drop Total) to help support hormone production in both men and women.

1 Drop Stress Away (TM) - Apply to wrists at night at bed time to help encourage more restful sleep

1 Life 5 (TM) (or other high quality probiotic) Probiotic – 1 Life 5 (TM) (or other high quality probiotic) Probiotic at night before bed

Level 3 AM:

2 Oz Ningxia Red – with 8 Oz of water (either drink it straight or add to water, but be sure to have water with it to increase its benefits).

1 Drop Lemon Oil – Add to 16 Oz of water and drink in the first few hours of your day.

1 Drop Fennel Oil – Apply over pancreas before 2 biggest meals throughout the day to help support

Normal pancreatic and insulin function.

1 Scoop Alka-Lime (TM) – To help manage body PH more efficiently and create a healing environment in the

Body. Can be mixed with Ningxia Red or drank separately with 8 Oz of water.

1 Drop EndoFlex (TM) – Apply one drop over thyroid, kidneys, pancreas, or under throat vitaflex point under

Big toe in the morning.

1 Drop Idaho Blue Spruce – Apply 1 drop total to insides of ankles in the AM to help support hormones.

1 Life 5 (TM) (or other high quality probiotic) Probiotic – Take one capsule in AM to help support a healthy intestinal flora and maximize nutrient absorption.

Level 3 Pre Workout:

1 Drop/Swipe Valor (TM) – 5 minutes before lift - applied to chest in clockwise circular motion to drive in.

1 Oz Ningxia Red – 5 minutes before lift either straight or in 8 Oz of water to help energize the body and sustain exercise longer.

1 Drop Peppermint – In 1 Oz of water and drink immediately before lift to get yourself fired up and energized further.

1 Drop Motivation TM (blend) – Apply one drop to wrists, rub for 10 seconds, and then inhale for 30 seconds immediately before workout.

1 Drop Balsam Fir – Apply one drop to chest immediately before workout – and to sore muscles as desired throughout the day.

Level 3 During Workout:

Mix all 4 in 32 Oz of water and consume during workout:

1 Drop Slique (TM) Essence – Helps support metabolism and hunger levels, as well as tastes and smells good.

1 Drop Grapefruit Oil – Helps support metabolism, and the smell alone can increase metabolism and help decrease hunger. Also aids in detoxification, especially in problematic cellulite areas, and can help assist in the buffering and recycling of Lactic Acid (the byproduct that makes you sore).

1 Drop Lime – Also supports digestion and circulatory system, overall body detoxification, and can help support the metabolism.

1 Drop Lemongrass – Helps detoxify and support the lymphatic system.

Level 3 Post Workout:

1 Drop Ocotea – Hold under tongue for 30 seconds then swallow, and enjoy your favorite post-workout shake/meal (Slique (TM) Bar/Green Smoothie!).

1 Drop Idaho Blue Spruce – Apply to insides of ankles at night (One Drop Total) to help support hormone production in both men and women.

1 Drop Stress Away (TM) - Apply to wrists at night at bed time to help encourage more restful sleep.

1 Life 5 (TM) (or other high quality probiotic) Probiotic – 1 Life 5 (TM) (or other high quality probiotic) Probiotic at night before bed.

1 Pill Thyromin (TM) – Take before bed to help support thyroid function.

CONNECT WITH ADAM RINGHAM

adam@get-oiled-up.com

Facebook

www.Facebook.com/GetOiledUp

On The Web

www.get-oiled-up.com

Contact us for bulk discounts on book copies

About The Author

Having spent over 11 years with Adam has easily spent more life living than most people actually live. I've had the pleasure to see him soar as a person as of late. His kind generosity, his always positive, always optimistic personality, is by far one of his best qualities. He's a self-educated man. You won't find letters behind his name, or titles hanging on his wall. I've met people with so many educational backgrounds and titles that can't hold a candle to show Adam's depth and knowledge in not only health, fitness, and essential oils, but mental health, body systems, theories, etc. He is a wealth of information and his love for learning only drives him to be better every day. This however; has not always been the case.

Adam's life has been one big ball of hyper activity. I suppose one would give him the title of an ADHD child to the max. He's always been very intelligent, but lacked focus, empathy, Motivation TM (blend), and a drive. Adam went to college, never earned a degree, and lived the typical college lifestyle; binge drinking, eating empty carbs, and going to the gym with his buddies. Two years into his college career he was called to active duty (having been a part of the Army National Guard) after 9/11 happened. He had 36 hours to drop out of school and get ready to leave for an extended period of time. Then upon return he didn't really feel the love for nursing school anymore (not to mention because of his extended time away he would have had to restart from square one). I think he knew deep down he had a higher calling to help people in different ways.

Adam and I married, but this was not without its struggles as well. Helping Adam deal with some PTSD, ADHD, excessive binge drinking turned alcoholism, unhealthy lifestyle habits (Adam did hit over 300lbs from this muscular beef cake I first met), and overall daily functioning took a toll on me and our marriage. Through the introduction of essential oils, counseling, and lots of communication repair we somehow made it through. We just celebrated our 9 year anniversary mark (with a baby due any day to boot)! I believe none of this would have come to be without Adam's determination to learn everything about the chemical aspects of oils, the brain and body functions, and how to mold the two together in a healthy way. He's a researcher of EVERYTHING. There isn't a subject he won't entertain. He's chosen to be more proactive with his life and our family's life - and he's a completely changed person because of it.

If you're ready to make a change or need to educate yourself on small healthy lifestyle changes this book is sure to do it. It's not about going to the gym and smashing it every day or eating low carbs, being the skinniest or the buffest, etc. It's about using the tools already out there to help you get the most out of your healthy lifestyle and routine. It will give you tips on how best to use oils in conjunction with a healthy workout schedule and a healthy "diet."

Kari Christensen (Ringham)

Wife to the Alkaline Alchemist (aka Adam Ringham)